WOMEN with ADHD, a radical guide.

Break Through Barriers,Stay Active and Embrace Neurodiversity

By John G. Ben

Introduction

There is little information on how attention deficit hyperactivity disorder (ADHD) specifically affects adult women. The subjects of study are more frequently men, children, and teenagers. Studies even in young toddlers reveal that guys are diagnosed correctly more frequently than girls.

These disparities may be caused by gender prejudice and underappreciated ADHD symptoms. Compared to boys, girls often exhibit less "hyperactive" behavior. The majority of research tends to concentrate heavily on the hyperactive ADHD characteristics that are more prevalent in guys. ADHD symptoms in young females who are not treated may worsen throughout adulthood. ADHD can lower your overall quality of life if it is not treated.

TABLE OF CONTENTS

CHAPTER 1

ADHD IN WOMEN

ADHD can manifest differently in ladies than it does in males in terms of symptoms. Females with ADHD are more prone to inattention than males with the disorder, who often exhibit greater rates of hyperactivity and impulsivity. This involves having trouble starting or finishing work, paying attention to details, or adhering to directions.

Girls and women may have different ADHD symptoms, and some people don't identify their condition until they are older and experiencing difficulties at work, at home, or in relationships.

How Females' ADHD Differs

A neurodevelopmental condition called ADHD is characterized by excessive impulsivity, hyperactivity, and inattention.

There are three forms of ADHD, according to the Diagnostic and Statistical Manual of Mental Disorders published by the American Psychiatric Association.

mostly absent-minded kind

mostly impulsive and hyperactive kind

Variety kind (where both inattentive and hyperactive-impulsive symptoms are present)

Although women with ADHD can have symptoms anywhere along this continuum, they are more frequently identified with the mainly inattentive variety of the disorder. For why this is, there are several physiological and psychological hypotheses.

The fact that the hippocampus is typically bigger in females than in males may have something to do with it. The hippocampus is susceptible to damage or impairment from a wide range of drugs or stimuli but plays a significant role in learning and memory.

The hippocampus of females has more estrogen receptors than that of males. These are cellular triggers that estrogen, a hormone found in females, activates. This is crucial since a woman's hormone changes may have a significant impact on how her brain works and may even hasten the emergence of ADHD symptoms.

The symptoms of ADHD in females may be further complicated by sociocultural factors. These include poor self-esteem and underachievement sentiments, which frequently start in infancy but can linger long into adulthood. As a result, inattentive symptoms may go unrecognized, in part because females' expectations diverge from guys' expectations frequently.

Because girls are frequently encouraged to bury their emotions rather than lashing out like boys, depression and anxiety are also more prevalent among females with ADHD. Females with ADHD may be affected by these gender norms just as much as by the condition itself.

Who Is Prone to ADHD?

Despite the widespread belief that men experience ADHD more frequently than women, recent evidence indicates that women are underdiagnosed with the disorder (in part because inattention is less disruptive than hyperactivity and impulsivity). If so, it may be closer than previously believed that women and men had similar rates of ADHD.

Common signs of inattentive ADHD in women include:

being criticized for negligent actions repeatedly

inability to handle many connections or multiple tasks

ignoring due dates

Putting off doing things till the last minute and procrastinating

"Spacing out" during meetings or conversations A problem with organization or cleanliness at work, home, or school.

Losing or misplacing items like your phone or spectacles on a regular basis

Frequently forgetting appointments or phone calls

difficulty making choices or developing workable plans

Although impulsive and hyperactive symptoms are less frequent in females with ADHD, they can nonetheless show themselves as:

Anxiety and fidgeting

Talking too much and changing topics or tasks frequently

Talking over or constantly interrupting others

difficulty relaxing or sitting still with others

difficulty sustaining friendships

In contrast to males, females frequently exhibit ADHD in distinct ways. Inattentional symptoms are more prevalent in girls and women than hyperactivity or impulsiveness.

Due to the fact that their symptoms are often less bothersome, females with ADHD are also more prone to sadness and anxiety and are typically identified later in life.

Women are taken ADHD medications less frequently than men because their symptoms are either overlooked or incorrectly diagnosed, even though the therapy for ADHD is the same for both genders (or because some people consider ADHD a predominantly male disease).

CHAPTER 2

COMMON ADHD SYMPTOMS

You might believe that males are more likely to have Attention Deficit/Hyperactivity Disorder (ADHD) than other age groups. Although it is frequently ignored or misunderstood, the National Institute of Mental Health says that 3.2% of American women between the ages of 18 and 44 have ADHD. It's crucial to empower yourself with accurate knowledge in this situation, especially if you're observing any ADHD symptoms or indicators.

What symptoms of female ADHD are there?

ADHD is diagnosed in men almost two times more frequently than in women. A research from King's College in London found that the disease might manifest in men as negative conduct, hyperactivity, difficulty focusing, and learning issues. Cook notes that among females who were assigned a gender at birth, "inattentive signs, not hyperactive symptoms, are what we find." Particularly, typical symptoms of ADHD in females include:

Making errors due to a lack of attention to detail

difficulty focusing and listening to others

difficulty with directions

being easily distracted

Forgetfulness

According to Ben, "We don't really understand why there is a gender split with ADHD symptoms." "It could have to do with socialization; girls are frequently taught from a young age not to cause trouble. There could possibly be a hereditary component, but further research is required to determine that for sure.

What effects may ADHD have on a woman's life?

A lady with ADHD may experience a variety of difficulties in her daily life. According to Dr. Goodman, women with undiagnosed ADHD routinely exhibit uneven task completion. Running late, missing appointments, losing your phone or keys, or being late picking up your kids from school are all examples of this. However, if you occasionally forget to pay a payment, it doesn't necessarily indicate that you have ADHD. Instead, you can identify signs of ADHD throughout your life.

It is beneficial for women with ADHD to recognize a persistent trend, according to Dr. Cook. Look back and see if symptoms like a lack of attention have harmed your life if they don't appear abruptly, such as after striking your head in a vehicle accident.

You may have heard the terms "erratic" or "unreliable" a lot too often. Dr. Goodman continues, "Women with ADHD may frequently not even be aware that they have a curable illness. "They could decide that "This is just who I am" after having to endure criticism for many years. It can be difficult to interrupt the loop of this sort of thinking, which can lead to sadness and poor self-esteem.

What should you do if you believe you may have ADHD?

A diagnosis is essential. You'll realize that what you have, ADHD, is separate from who you are as a person once your symptoms have been successfully controlled, according to Dr. Goodman. "Your confidence level will increase. The best method to get a thorough evaluation is to see a medical professional who has knowledge of and experience treating individuals with ADHD. A thorough examination involves a long list of questions to examine the presence or absence of numerous mental diseases beyond just ADHD because 70% of individuals with ADHD also have another psychiatric condition.

Medication and therapy are the two primary methods of treating ADHD. Medication is frequently used as the first line of treatment for ADHD in both children and adults, occasionally in conjunction with counseling.

Medication

Medication usage is lower in girls and women than in boys and men with ADHD, although this is more a result of underdiagnosis and biased treatment referrals than it is because it is because it is more effective.

Although they won't completely cure your ADHD, medications can help make your symptoms easier to control. The two most often used psychostimulants for treating ADHD are amphetamines (such as Adderall and Vyvanse) and methylphenidate (such as Concerta, Focalin, Focalin XR, Daytrana, and Metadate).

Drugs used as psychostimulants aim to control the brain chemicals that influence behavior and attention.

Additionally, non-stimulant medications including guanfacine, clonidine, and strattera are available. Due to the numerous hazards associated with using stimulants to treat ADHD, Thriveworks doctors and nurse practitioners do not recommend them. When stimulants are taken improperly, there is a substantial chance of misuse as well as a wide range of negative side effects, including high blood pressure, strokes, and seizures.

Counseling

It may be a mix of different therapy modalities that works best for you in order to address both co-occurring anxiety or depression and ADHD. In addition to talk therapy, other

ADHD-specific coaching may be beneficial for you, based on your unique situation and symptoms.

Learning effective coping mechanisms and life management techniques is the major goal since they will help you control your symptoms and possibly even improve your self-esteem.

Women with ADHD, in particular, can greatly benefit from the knowledge and support offered in talk therapy or support groups because anxiety and sadness so frequently coexist with their ADHD. Knowing that other people experience stress and rejection on an equal basis to you might be comforting.

CHAPTER 3

WHY WOMEN BATTLE ADHD MORE

Many females with ADHD don't receive a proper diagnosis until they are in their 30s. After their children are identified as having ADHD and they exhibit some of the symptoms themselves, parents frequently seek a diagnosis and therapy.

Here are some of the most significant factors that contribute to the underdiagnosis of ADHD in women.

ADHD is incorrectly understood

Despite efforts by supporters and experts to shift perceptions, ADHD is still a problem. Many individuals, even experts, still refer to ADHD as "hyperactive boys' disorder," whether they work as teachers or mental health professionals.

One reason women frequently go misdiagnosed in childhood is because adults aren't educated to identify all the symptoms of ADHD, particularly when it manifests in females.Since the majority of the research underlying the symptoms used to diagnose ADHD has been conducted on males, many crucial presentations may be being ignored.

ADHD: Hyperactive vs. inattentive

When it comes to the inattentive subtype of ADHD, women are more likely to exhibit. Instead of being hyperactive, people with this kind of ADHD are more prone to be easily distracted.

It makes sense that females with inattentive ADHD frequently go unnoticed when teachers and other adults exclusively focus on hyperactivity and restlessness as the only symptoms of the disorder. Consider this: Which child—the one calmly dozing at the back of the room or the one that is continuously rushing around and exhibiting bursts of energy—is more likely to get your attention?

Both in girls and in boys, signs of inattentive ADHD are frequently overlooked. Girls may not exhibit any hyperactivity at all (or may work harder to conceal it), which makes it difficult for people to detect them.

Boys "act out," while girls "act in."

Girls internalize their ADHD symptoms more than guys do.

Boys with ADHD may act out when they encounter difficulties. For instance, they can refuse to do the assignment or act defiantly toward parents and professors.

They are therefore more prone to vent their anger in public. They may get into "trouble" at school or at home as a result, but they also receive the desired attention.

Conversely, girls are more inclined to internalize their emotions. They could put the blame on themselves for their inability to do things that come naturally to their classmates. They could describe themselves as "ditzy" or "dumb."This doesn't get attention, and it also makes emotional anguish for females with ADHD worse.

There is little question that gender stereotypes and the expectations placed on women in society have a role in the gender disparity in ADHD diagnoses.

Women and girls could "conceal" symptoms.

Girls and women are typically expected to have it all together, whether it's overt or covert. Women are expected to keep things organized and to know where everything belongs, both at home and at work. They must conduct themselves and definitely refrain from having fits of rage or excessive energy.

In order to "hide" their symptoms, girls and women with ADHD learn how to do so.

The word "masking" refers to the coping mechanisms that persons with ADHD learn to employ in order to disguise their symptoms and blend in. For instance, they could quit talking out loud for the sake of not saying "enough." In an effort to prevent being late, they could start showing up to activities really early. When done frequently, masking may be quite draining and even distressing.

But as the saying goes, the grease goes to the squeaky wheel. Girls and women are less likely to receive the assistance and attention they require if they conceal their ADHD symptoms.

Getting Women's ADHD Treatment

It's likely that you had a challenging upbringing attempting to manage your symptoms on your own if you are a woman with ADHD. However, it doesn't have to be this way. With the appropriate diagnosis, you can have access to a successful therapy that can greatly simplify

your life.

Why women should seek therapy for ADHD

Other emotional and mental health issues like sadness, anxiety, and poor self-esteem are more prevalent among women with ADHD. This could be because women often aren't diagnosed until they are adults. This implies that women frequently spend their entire lives blaming themselves for what are basically merely symptoms of ADHD and not true "shortcomings."

You may arm yourself with the tools you need to live successfully with ADHD by receiving a diagnosis and receiving treatment. Additionally, it might comfort you that you're not sluggish, slow, or dim that certain things appear harder for you than they do for others. It's not your fault that you have ADHD; you simply do.

CHAPTER 4

TIME MANAGEMENT AND ADHD

Adults with attention deficit hyperactivity disorder (ADHD) frequently exhibit restlessness, impulsivity, and difficulty focusing. Additionally, their perspectives on time diverge. An inability to adequately prepare, an extraordinary capacity for procrastination, and an inability to tune out the noise around them are all characteristics that make it difficult to meet deadlines or even simply arrive on time. We examine time management difficulties for individuals with ADHD in this post and provide Several suggestions for improvement.

We sympathize if time management is a struggle for you. If you have adult ADHD (or believe that you have), your struggles may be made even more difficult by the overwhelming and chaotic nature of life.

What Are the Time Management Challenges Associated with ADHD?

The difficulties that come with ADHD are immense. Simple daily chores might quickly become difficult. A few of the symptoms of ADHD that can cause problems in daily life include hyperactivity, difficulty focusing, and interrupting others. The hardest problem of all is frequently time management, which includes learning how to manage time itself as well as getting things done on time.

Adults with ADHD: Time Management Advice

When it comes to managing your time and, by implication, controlling your adult ADHD, you have a variety of effective tools at your disposal. These strategies can help you remain on track and complete any chores that come your way, even if you just have moderate ADHD.

1. Use a calendar

Organizing your schedule by adding all of your appointments to a calendar is an excellent place to start. Whether it's a physical calendar, a smartphone app, or a day planner, keep it in one place and check it frequently, ideally at the same time each day.

2. Make a daily to-do list.

Making a master list is an essential first step in overcoming ADHD symptoms. Establish the practice of writing down your morning goals on a list. Keep this list as realistic as possible so that you have a probability of doing everything on it. Check off each assignment as you finish it!

3. Use your phone to set reminders

Your smartphone may be a great tool to help you stay focused and on track throughout the day in addition to a paper planner. Reminders are a useful tool for reminding oneself to do activities, and they may be configured in countless ways. Even better, you could program your alarm to remind you to "Check Calendar."

4. Set Task Priorities

Prioritizing your chores is something you should do after making your planner and setting your reminders. Choose an approach that works best for you—numbers or letters—and stick with it. Make sure to prioritize chores in order of importance, then move on to things that can wait until later.

5. Dividing tasks into 15-minute segments

The best method to turn what seems like a mountain into something that is actually doable is to divide your calendar into 15-minute halves. It is simpler to complete one task and then move on to the next in 15-minute increments.

6. Use a calendar application.

Utilizing calendar applications is an excellent method to prevent your ADHD from taking over. A calendar app will constantly remind you of the things you could otherwise easily forget since everyone always has their phone with them.

7. Put your necessities in order so you won't forget them.

Nobody understands the struggle more than folks with ADHD when they want to leave the house but can't find their keys. Create secure locations where items will always be to make it hard to lose or misplace them: a hook for your keys, a designated nook for your wallet, a visible spot for your notepad. You'll never again lose crucial objects if you concentrate on repetition when putting them in the same location.

8. Define timing (To Understand How Much Time Tasks Take)

Adults with ADHD frequently see time passing differently. Timers may be used to assign tasks certain amounts of time and notify you when that time is over. Consider setting an alarm that goes off at regular intervals for lengthier work. Utilizing timers ultimately aims to help you comprehend how long each action truly takes by bringing your senses into alignment with the passage of time.

9. Position clocks so that you can see them.

Time blindness, or a lack of awareness of the passing of time, is a prevalent issue among many individuals with ADHD, and analog clocks can help you combat it. Hearing a clock's ticking can occasionally be helpful for keeping track of time as well as for pacing and timing tasks.

10. Double the time you anticipate it will take to complete each task. It

It's challenging to estimate how long a certain job will take when one is "blind" to the passing of time. One of the greatest methods is to estimate how long the work will take, then double (or even treble) that time to increase the window of opportunity for completion. This will make it simpler for you to plan in the future by helping you know for sure how long a given job will take.

11. Stick Post-It Notes Everywhere

It's best if you allow yourself as many small cues as possible to stay on track with your goals. Sticky notes externalize a vital process that ADHD can make occasionally too challenging to control, making it simple to duplicate the notes that ought to be in your head.

You may have ADHD if time management is a problem for you. Klarity is here to assist you in locating the best physician, whether you need a diagnostic or a course of treatment. Set up your 30-minute online appointment with a doctor right away to get started on the path to a more organized and content future.

CHAPTER 5

HOW TO ACCEPT AND EMBRACE YOUR ADHD

Your relationship with yourself is the most significant one you will ever have.

Valentine's Day appears to highlight the idea that love is, in fact, a mystery every year. Some people anxiously anticipate this day since it will be their time to show their love for individuals they care about or get love in return. However, for many adults with ADHD, their internal battle with low self-esteem, a lack of acceptance of who they are, and a lack of value prevents them from fully appreciating the bountiful love they get from others around them and from themselves.

ADHD in Adults and Low Self-Esteem

It is nearly impossible to appreciate your own natural talents and innate value, let alone share and receive this joy with others, when you have spent your entire life trying to live up to other people's expectations and your mind is filled with self-sabotaging thoughts. Unfortunately, a lot of people with ADHD hide by themselves behind feelings of self-blame, shame, emptiness, disappointment, sadness, and passion. I hope that on this Valentine's Day, people with ADHD will give themselves the respect they deserve and recognize the heart they bring to the world.

Hopefully, the advice provided below may enable each of us to feel a little more pleased, joyful, and appreciative of ourselves.

Release the past

You merit a new beginning! Everyone has experienced obstacles that have made life difficult, if not occasionally impossible. Don't exclude yourself from the prospect of a prosperous future because of failures in the past, misunderstandings, or the mistrust or ignorance of others. Put the emotions and circumstances that lead you to this point in time behind you after acknowledging them. Finally make the choice to not carry these wounds and regrets into the future.

Accept Yourself

You have undoubtedly already made up for your past mistakes. Stop punishing and mistreating yourself by clinging to this error. You are not serving anybody by continuing in this manner, and it is keeping you from moving on with your life. Instead, consider the lessons you have taken away from this event. Sometimes the only things we can learn from our errors are the new skills we developed and the determination to never repeat them. Delete it...

If You Don't Have Nice Things To Say

The proverb "If you can't say something pleasant, don't say anything at all" is one that most people have heard. You should consider this as well. Many of us still talk down to ourselves in front of other people or let our inner critic speak negatively about us. Stop talking negatively about yourself or giving in to the nagging, gloomy ideas that keep popping up in your brain. Everybody has inner critics or "gremlins" that constantly undermine their own confidence by asking questions like, "How could you be so stupid? " Nothing you try to accomplish is proper. … What do you think of yourself? … "You'll never get it properly," the speaker said. Be aware that you may lessen these negative ideas by first being aware of them, at which point you can tell your inner critic, "If you can't offer anything kind...

Take Initiative

Make sure to go closer to your greater dreams every day by taking tiny measures. You may advance on your trip by taking even baby steps in the correct way. On certain days, all you need to do is jot down five positive traits about yourself. On other days, it can include making a more thorough strategy to realize a certain desire or devoting more time to actually accomplishing the tasks on your "to do" list. You may achieve success by taking little, deliberate measures.

Enjoy Yourself Laugh aloud.

Amazing, intrinsic talents that people with ADHD possess sometimes go undiscovered and unutilized. It makes sense that you don't value yourself. We have been attempting to be someone else much too frequently. Be true to yourself! You possess a special set of abilities and gifts that are designed to be shared. Stop trying to be what other people have expected of you your entire life; it's not working anyhow. Smiling will arouse curiosity in others around you. Wear bare feet. Do something that makes you grin or laugh aloud. You should enjoy yourself, your life, your relationships, and your surroundings. This life is too full of wonder and beauty to not be appreciative of it. Spend time engaging in the activities that make you happy.

Being yourself

Amazing, intrinsic talents that people with ADHD possess sometimes go undiscovered and unutilized. It makes sense that you don't value yourself. We have been attempting to be someone else much too frequently. Be true to yourself! You possess a special set of abilities and gifts that are designed to be shared. Stop trying to be what other people have expected of you your entire life; it's not working anyhow.

You can start now to build the loving life you deserve,

so go ahead, let the past go, forgive yourself, take action, have fun, and be yourself. Happy Valentine's Day to you all, and may you all always remember how wonderful you are to the world.

Strengthening self-compassion

Self-compassion is a complimentary strategy that could enable all other aspects of ADHD treatment to advance. Making new goals and routines, adhering to them, and making adjustments to them are difficult when things go wrong. The key to resilient ADHD treatment is to be patient with errors, get yourself together, and move on.

Here is a drill for you: Imagine a challenging circumstance, or imagine yourself in one. Recognize whatever you are experiencing as you inhale each breath. This is a difficult time. Everyone has difficult times. Then, on each exhale, concentrate on making yourself whatever wish you would make for a buddy. May I have happiness, tranquility, or at least a reduction in my stress and suffering.

Don't worry about the exact wording, just concentrate on what feels right. Practice letting go of judgment and wanting for yourself what you would wish for a loved one or friend without pushing any specific emotion. Give yourself credit for whatever you've achieved, ADHD or not. Giving oneself some leeway does not imply that you are ideal as you are. You are excellent the way you are because that is who you are, but just like everyone else, you have room for improvement. Because of ADHD, decisions must be made that require time and effort. ADHD makes things tough. All of it is accurate, so accept your weaknesses, give attention to your talents, and then go on with confidence and compassion.

CHAPTER 6

TREATMENT FOR WOMEN

The suggested method for treating ADHD in women and girls takes into account each patient's unique needs, stage of life, and symptom intensity in addition to providing evidence-based medication and behavioral therapy.

A multimodal strategy is necessary for effective treatment, which frequently entails prescription drugs, therapy, counseling, stress-reduction methods, and modifications to one's environment at work and at home. To control their ADHD, some women and girls choose a variety of lifestyle measures.

The difficulty of getting the right care

Finding a doctor who can offer effective therapy for women with an ADHD diagnosis might be difficult. Even though the number of physicians skilled in treating adult ADHD is expanding, it can be challenging to locate a specialist who understands the difficulties women encounter when managing therapy. The majority of physicians employ traditional psychotherapy techniques, which can shed light on emotional and interpersonal problems but do not assist a woman with ADHD in learning how to better control the disease or acquire skills to lead a more fulfilling and productive life.

The stage of life that a woman or girl is at must be taken into account when managing their ADHD. Changes in hormone levels, duties at home, at work, or in school, relationships with significant others, partners, or spouses, and interactions with friends, coworkers, and family members can all have an impact on symptom levels. In order to manage ADHD symptoms and modify therapy to meet the unique requirements of a woman or girl, co-occurring illnesses must also be managed.

Self-esteem, interpersonal, and familial concerns, daily health routines, everyday stress levels, and life management skills are all addressed by ADHD-focused therapy. This type of intervention, which combines cognitive behavior therapy with cognitive rehabilitation procedures, is sometimes referred to as "neurocognitive psychotherapy." While the cognitive rehabilitation approach focuses on life management skills for improving cognitive functions (remembering, reasoning, understanding, problem solving, evaluating, and using judgment), learning compensatory strategies, and restructuring the environment, cognitive behavior therapy focuses on psychological issues related to ADHD (such as self-esteem, self-acceptance, and self-blame).

According to recent studies, untreated or poorly managed
ADHD symptoms are linked to both general health and life
expectancy. Poorly managed ADHD has a significant
impact on a person's capacity to control other chronic
medical illnesses including diabetes, high blood pressure,
or depression. This poor overall health management can
lead to conditions of persistent poor health and raise the
chance of an early death when combined with chronic
stress.

ADHD medication treatment

ADHD cannot be cured by medication. When it works, it
lessens the symptoms of ADHD while they are present in a
girl or woman's body. Medication falls basically into two
categories: stimulant and nonstimulant. Sometimes
doctors will give patients a drug off-label that wasn't
intended to treat ADHD but has been shown to lessen
some of its symptoms.

It might be trickier to prescribe drugs for women with
ADHD than it is for males. Throughout the menstrual cycle,
in relation to birth control or assisted reproductive
technologies, and at various life phases (such as puberty,
pregnancy, perimenopause, and menopause), hormone
variations can exacerbate ADHD symptoms, particularly
when estrogen levels are low.

When estrogen levels are fluctuating and declining the greatest in certain women approaching or in menopause, hormone replacement treatment may be paired with medicines for improved symptom control.

Every facet of a woman's life, including the management of coexisting illnesses, must be taken into account while developing a drug management strategy. Women with ADHD frequently have alcohol and drug use difficulties, particularly if the condition has gone untreated. Before writing a prescription, this necessitates taking a thorough history of substance usage. This stage is intended to assist the doctor and patient in selecting the medicine that is best suitable for the particular set of circumstances, not to discourage the use of pharmaceuticals in therapy.

Behavior modification for symptoms of ADHD

Along with medication management, behavioral or psychosocial counseling may be advised for females with ADHD. The importance of behavioral therapy for ADHD is multifaceted. First of all, females with ADHD experience issues in everyday life that go well beyond their symptoms, such as poor conduct and academic performance in school, strained relationships with siblings and friends, disobedience to authority figures, and strained connections with their parents. These issues are crucial because they indicate how long-term performance for kids with ADHD will be.

Once a girl or adolescent has been diagnosed with ADHD, behavioral therapies should begin right away. Effective behavioral therapy for children with ADHD shouldn't be delayed by parents, educators, or professionals.

Behavioral management for women will likely incorporate more lifestyle supports as well as CBT. A kind of mental health care called cognitive-behavioral therapy concentrates on the thoughts and actions that take place right now. This method is distinct from conventional psychoanalytic or psychodynamic therapy, which involves revisiting and reprocessing the early life events that may have contributed to contemporary emotional issues. CBT differs from these earlier therapies in that its objectives and strategies are made explicit and, as a result, are measurable for every patient.

For adults with ADHD, CBT treatments have been created expressly for them.

Some of these programs are designed to assist people in overcoming their challenges with daily executive functions, which are essential for time management, organization, and long- and short-term planning. Other programs concentrate on impulse control, stress management, and emotional self-regulation.

Despite not being expressly created to address the symptoms and impairments associated with ADHD, women who are using CBT for comorbid illnesses such as depression and anxiety may find this therapy useful for their ADHD symptoms.

Around 6 in 100 children and adolescents and 3 in 100 adults have ADHD, a common neurodevelopmental disease. The main signs of the disorder are impulsivity, hyperactivity, and inattentiveness. Additionally, it is linked to a number of comorbid diseases, social interaction issues, and other issues.

The DSM-5 may be used to diagnose ADHD, and depending on the fundamental symptoms that a person exhibits, there are three distinct presentation types.

The symptoms must have existed since childhood and for at least six months in more than one place. Similar criteria are anticipated to be present in ICD-11, the first version of this diagnostic system to recognize ADHD.

There has been a great deal of research on ADHD risk factors. Although genetic investigations have not yet shown a definite genetic basis for the illness, it is known to be highly heritable. Multiple genes are likely implicated, according to studies. There are environmental risk factors as well, and certain prenatal occurrences have been linked to an increased chance of ADHD.

The brain circuitry involved in selective attention, which includes parts like the prefrontal cortex and a variety of neurotransmitters but most importantly dopamine, is thought to be at the root of ADHD.

The age of the person affects how ADHD is managed. All ages can get psychosocial and biological therapies, although younger patients should use medicine with caution because it is unclear exactly what long-term consequences it will have on the growing brain.

www.ingramcontent.com/pod-product-compliance
Lightning Source LLC
Chambersburg PA
CBHW071029260726
48662CB00024B/2201